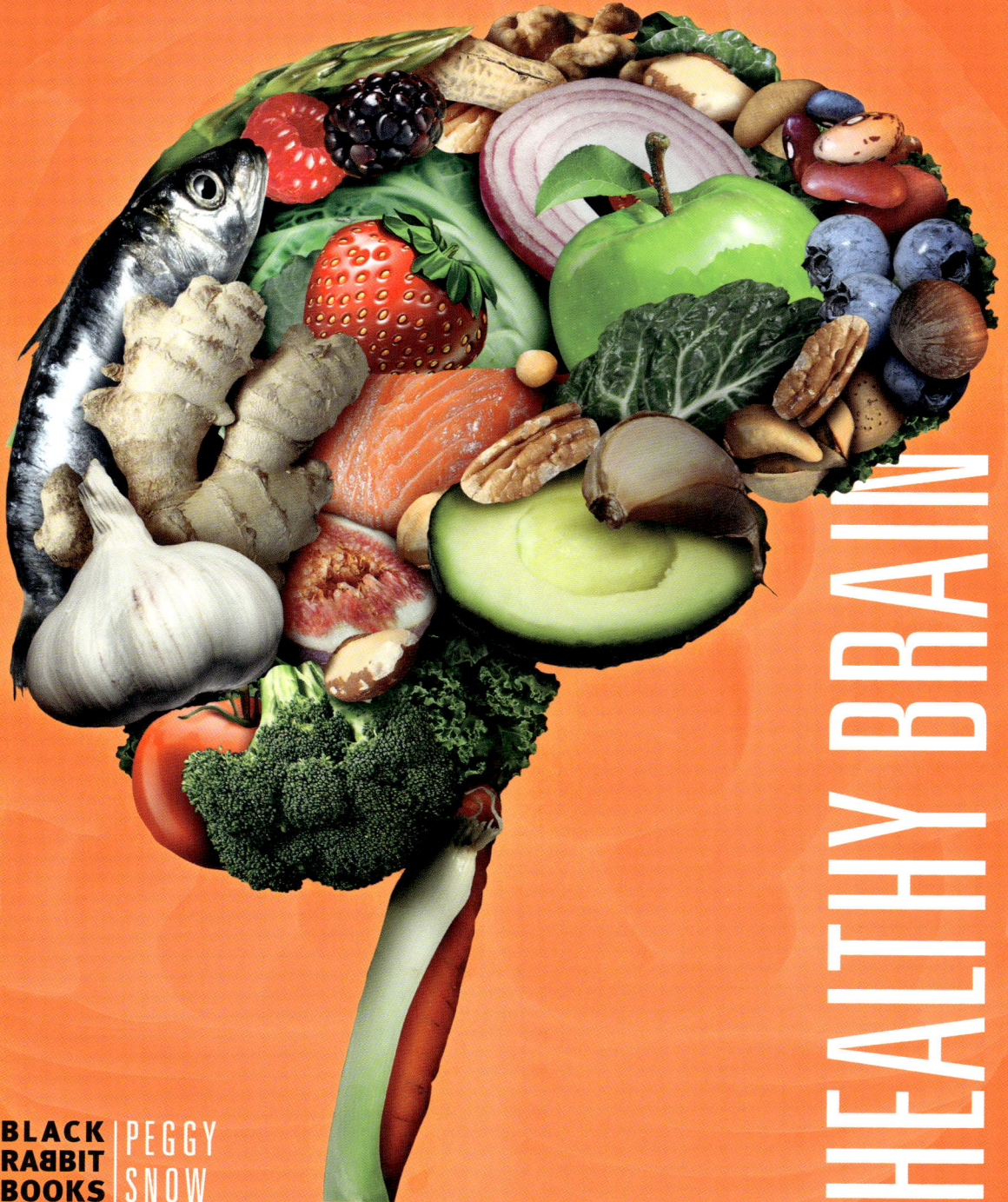

HEALTHY BRAIN

BLACK RABBIT BOOKS

PEGGY SNOW

TABLE OF CONTENTS

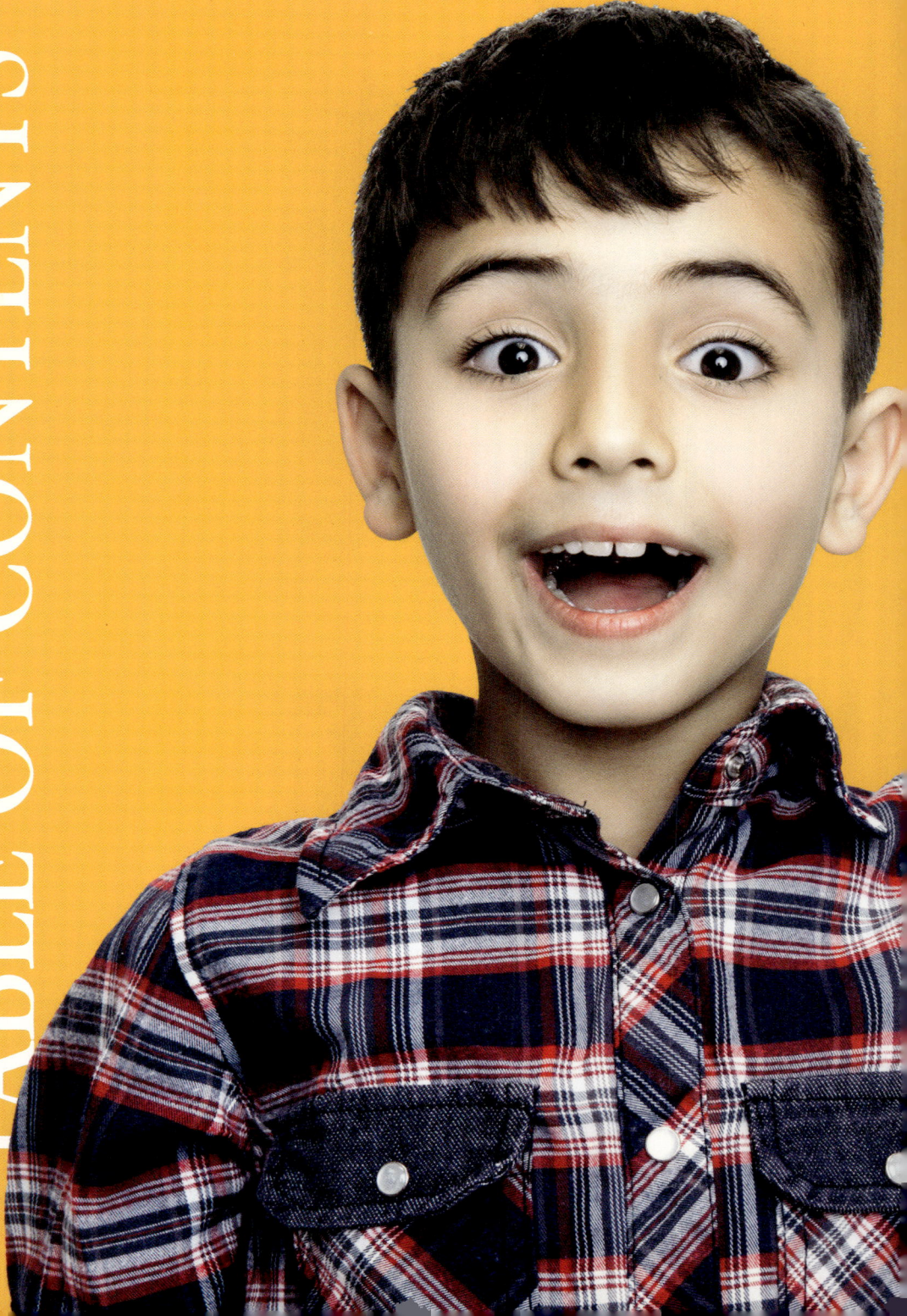

1. Use Your Senses   4

2. Be Active   6

3. Eat Healthy 10

4. Be Curious 13

5. Have Fun 16

6. Take a Break 19

More to Explore   22

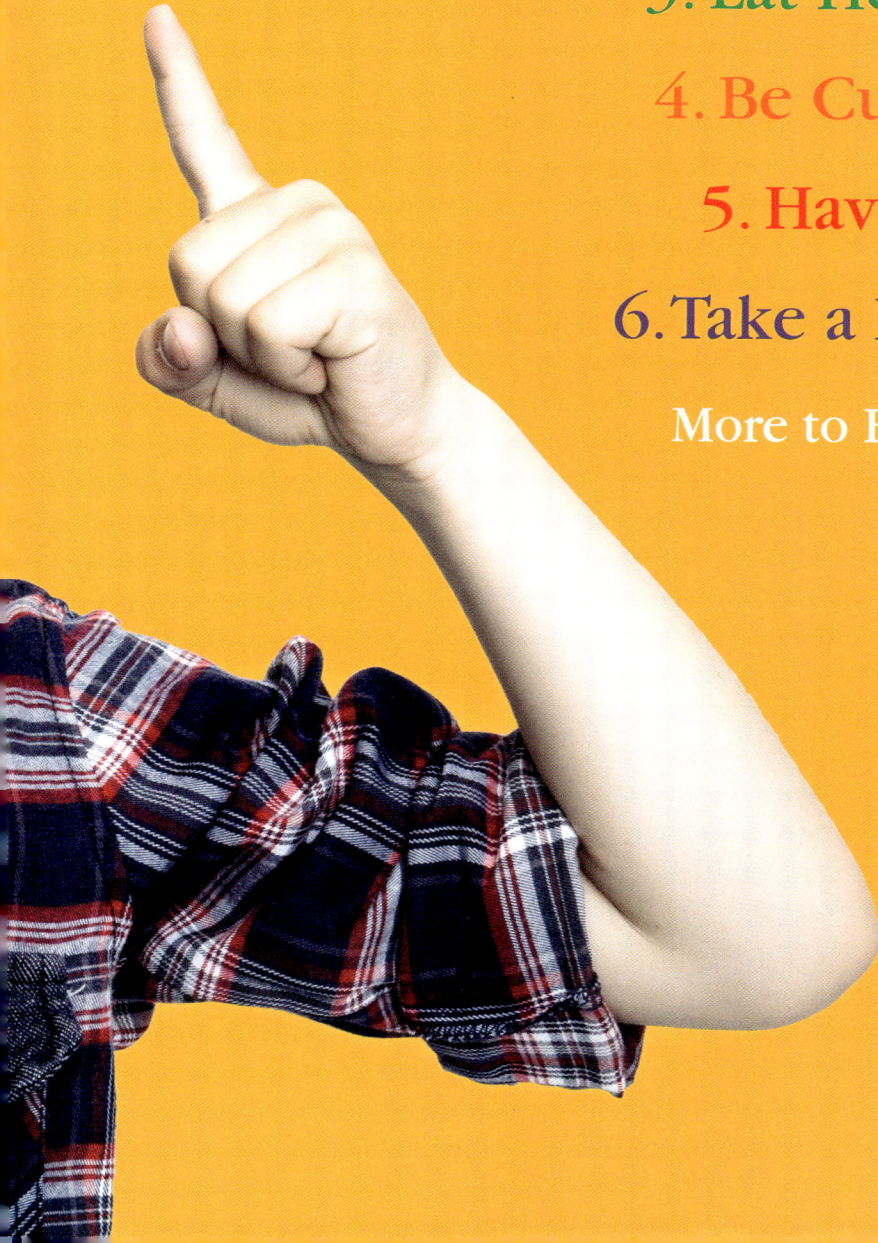

1

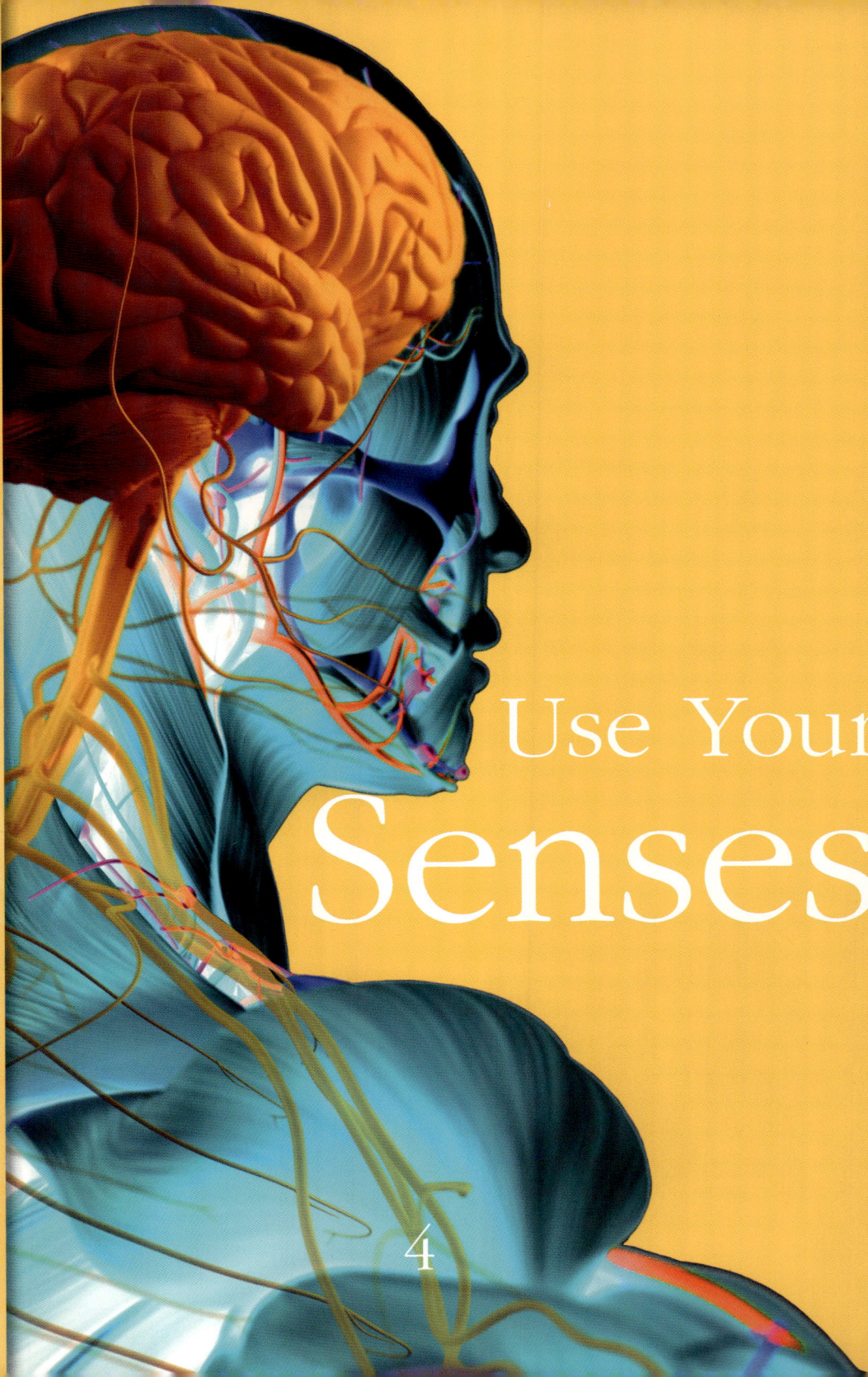

Use Your
Senses

4

Your brain is in charge of your body. This includes your senses. Your brain processes everything you see, hear, taste, smell, and touch. Your senses are learning helpers. Using them can make learning easier.

Using more than one sense at a time can help you learn. And it helps you remember. When your teacher reads aloud, you might look at pictures. You hear and see. Using cereal or beads can help with math. You see and touch.

Think About It
How many senses could you use for an art project?

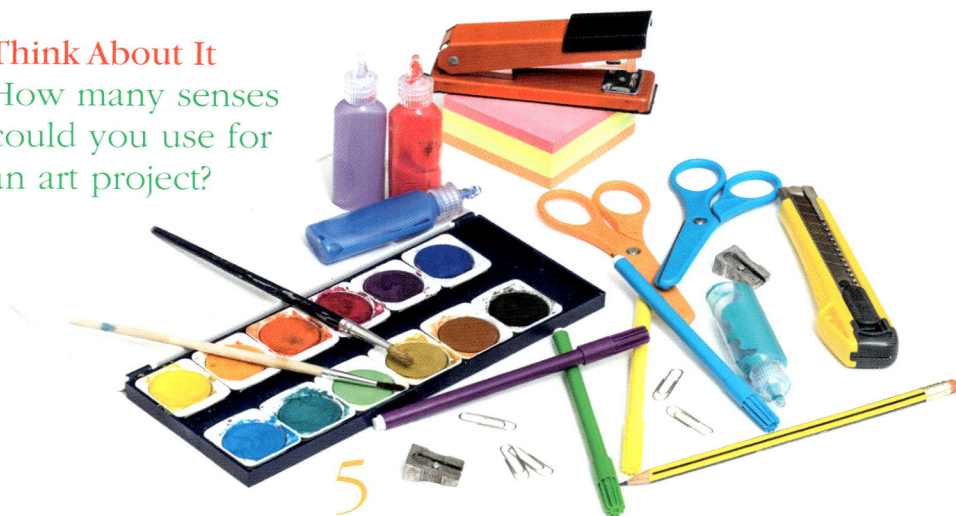

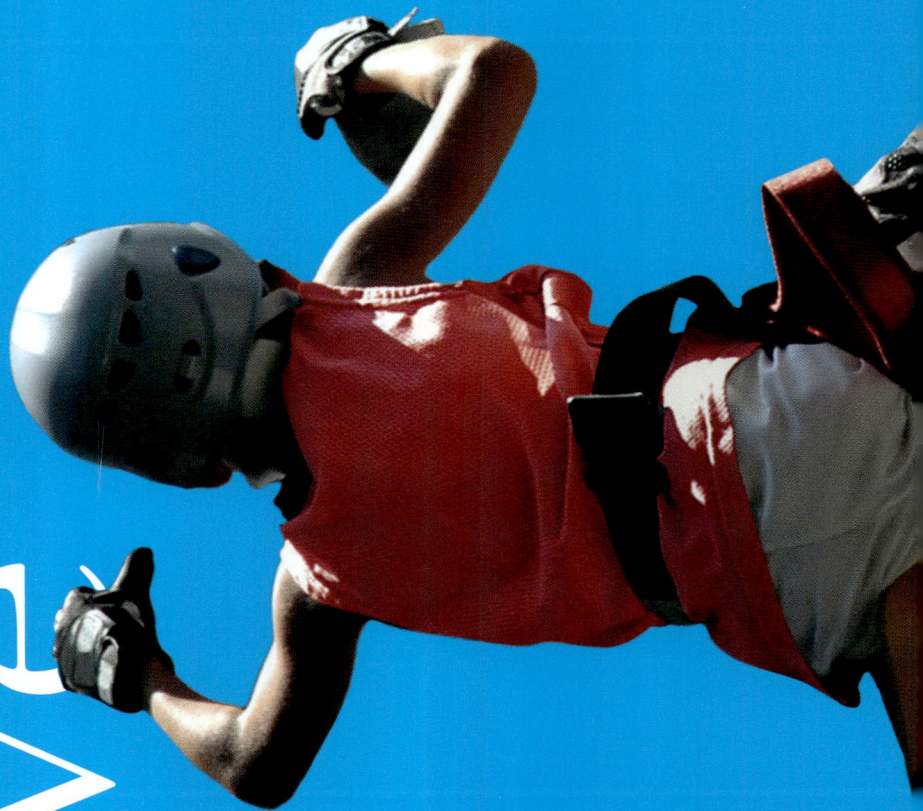

Be Active

2

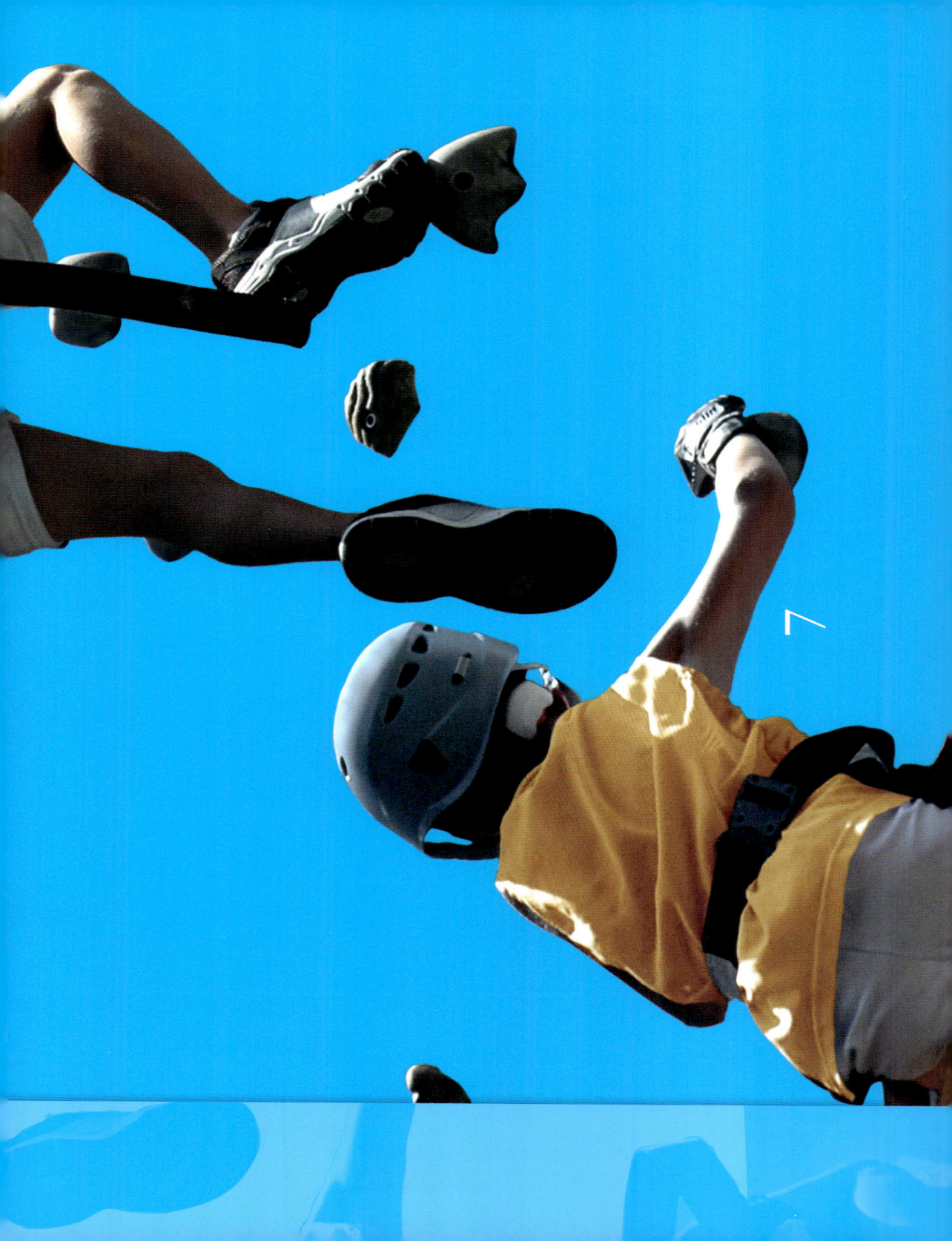

When you're active, your heart pumps more blood to your brain. Your brain gets more oxygen. You feel better and you think more clearly.

Being active helps you focus and learn. Your memory will improve too.

Playing kickball, jumping rope, and climbing can help you do better in school. So can any activity that gets your heart pumping.

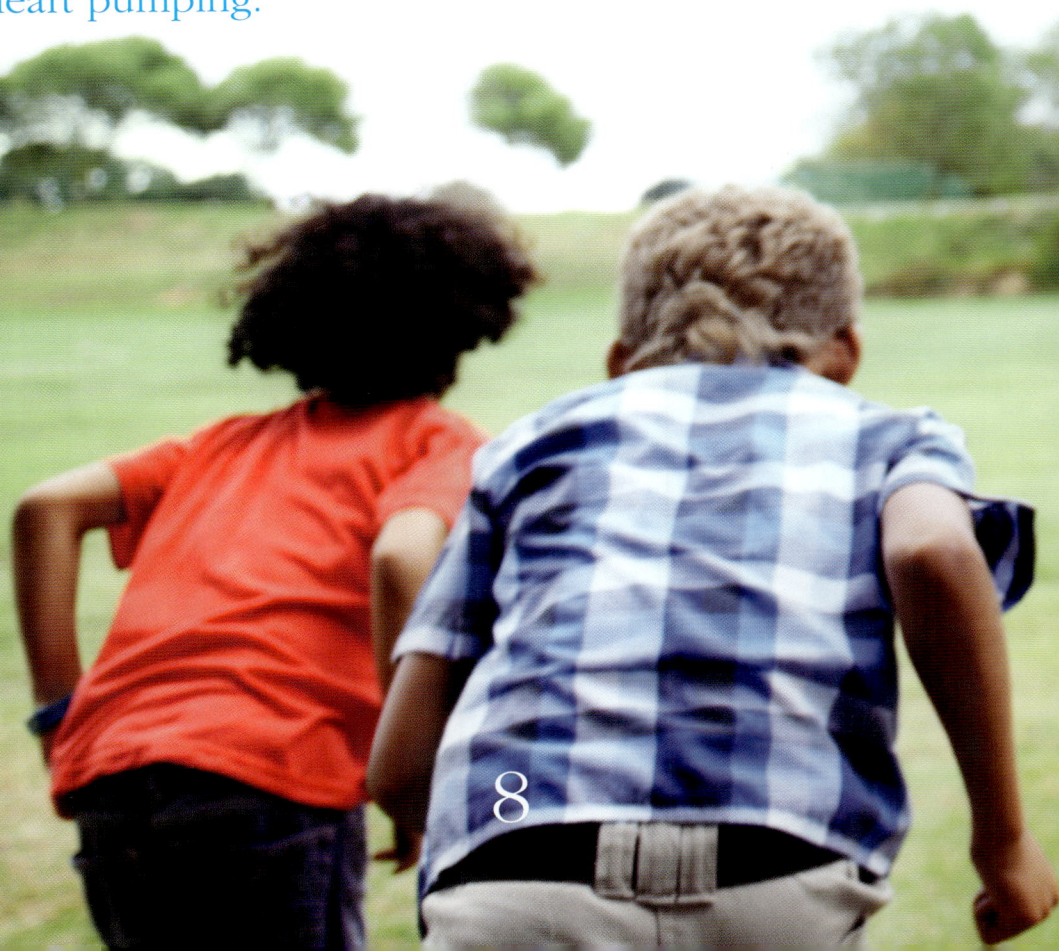

8

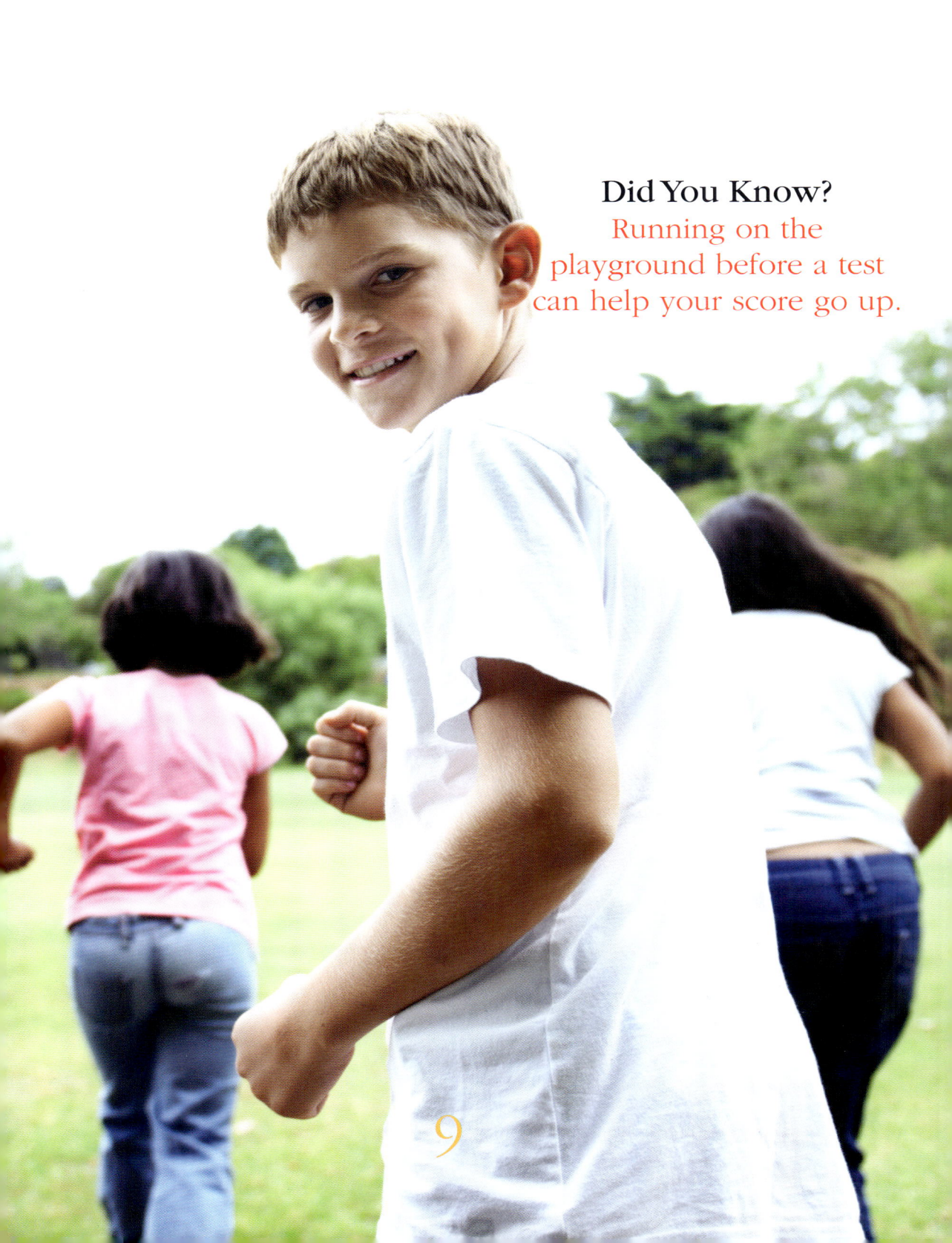

Did You Know?
Running on the playground before a test can help your score go up.

Eat
Healthy

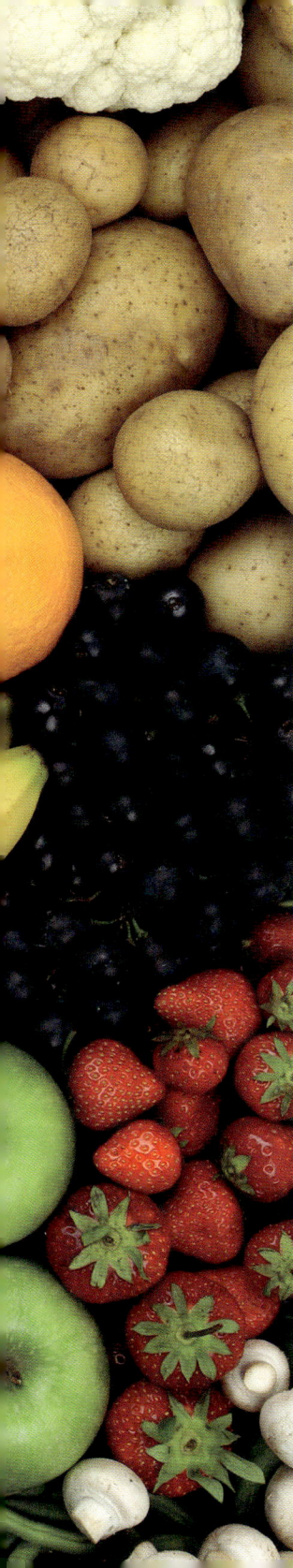

Your brain needs vitamins and minerals from healthy food. Many fruits and vegetables provide these. Spinach, carrots, and red peppers are good choices. So are bananas, strawberries, and oranges.

Dairy foods like milk and cottage cheese are healthy. Oatmeal gives you fiber. Eggs, beans, and chicken give you protein.

Eating healthy food helps you think clearly, learn, and remember.

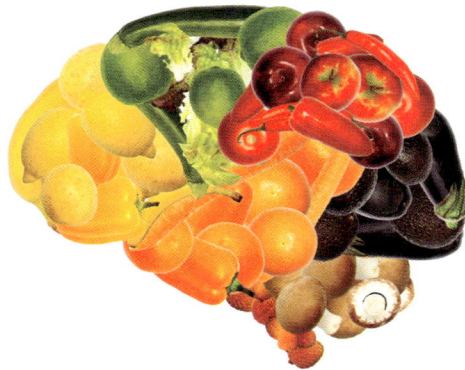

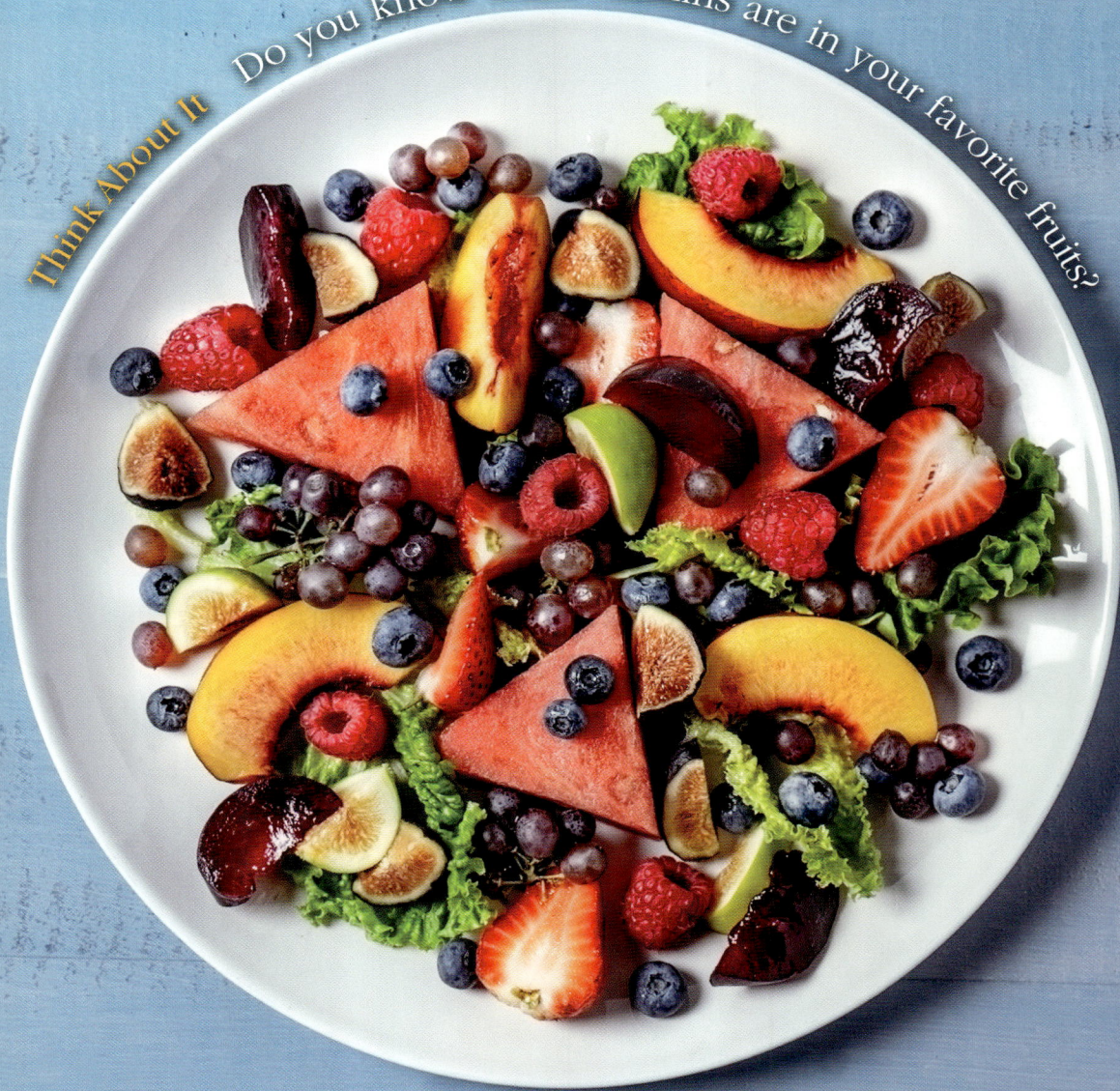

12

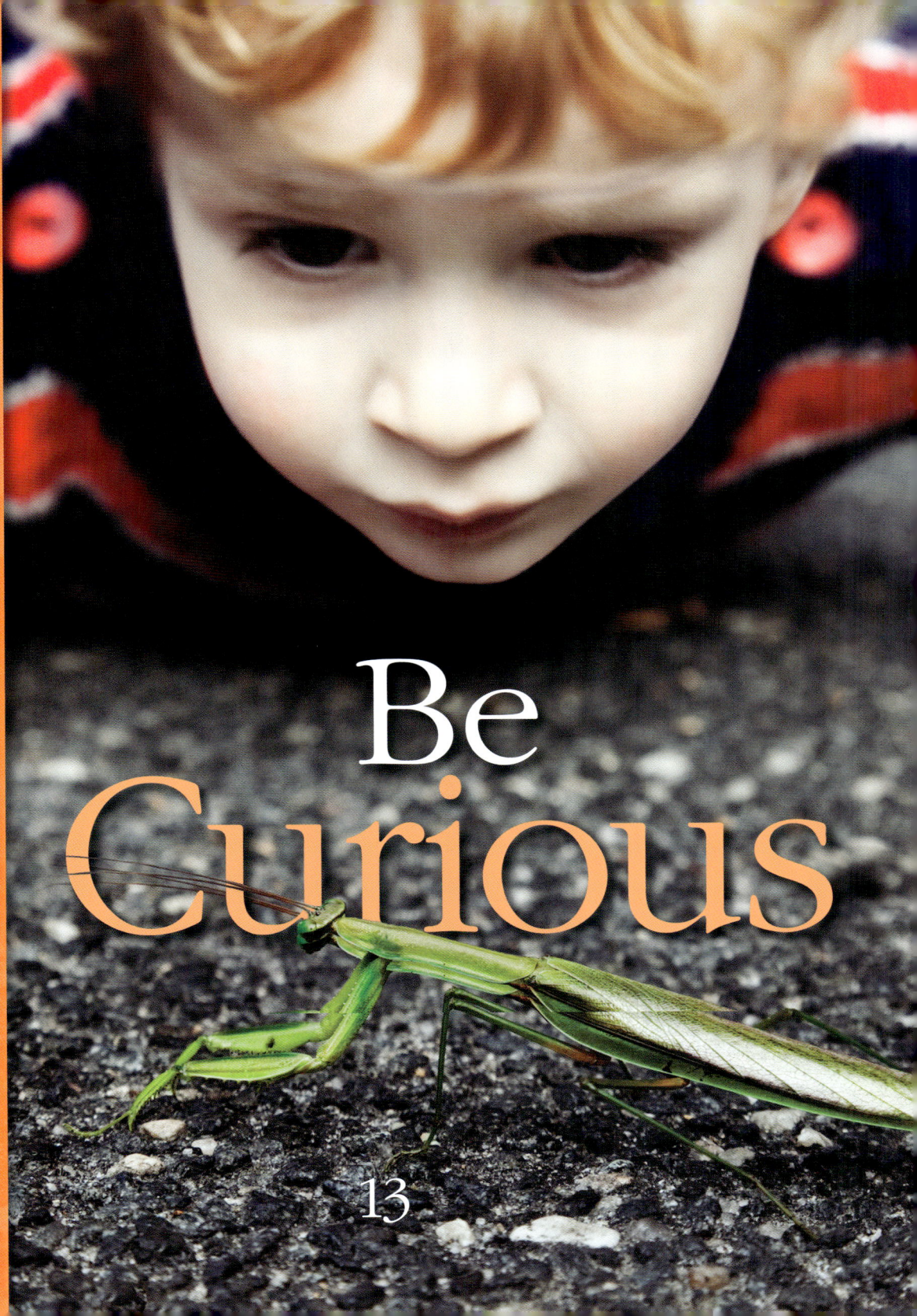

Be Curious

Being curious is good exercise for your brain. It improves your thinking skills. When you're curious, you wonder about things. You ask questions.

You might wonder, "What are clouds? Why is the sky blue? How do fish breathe?" You can read to find answers. Reading can lead to more curiosity.

You can be curious and active at the same time. Go on a nature walk. Take a close look at the bugs and plants. Or visit a museum. Some museums let you learn and play.

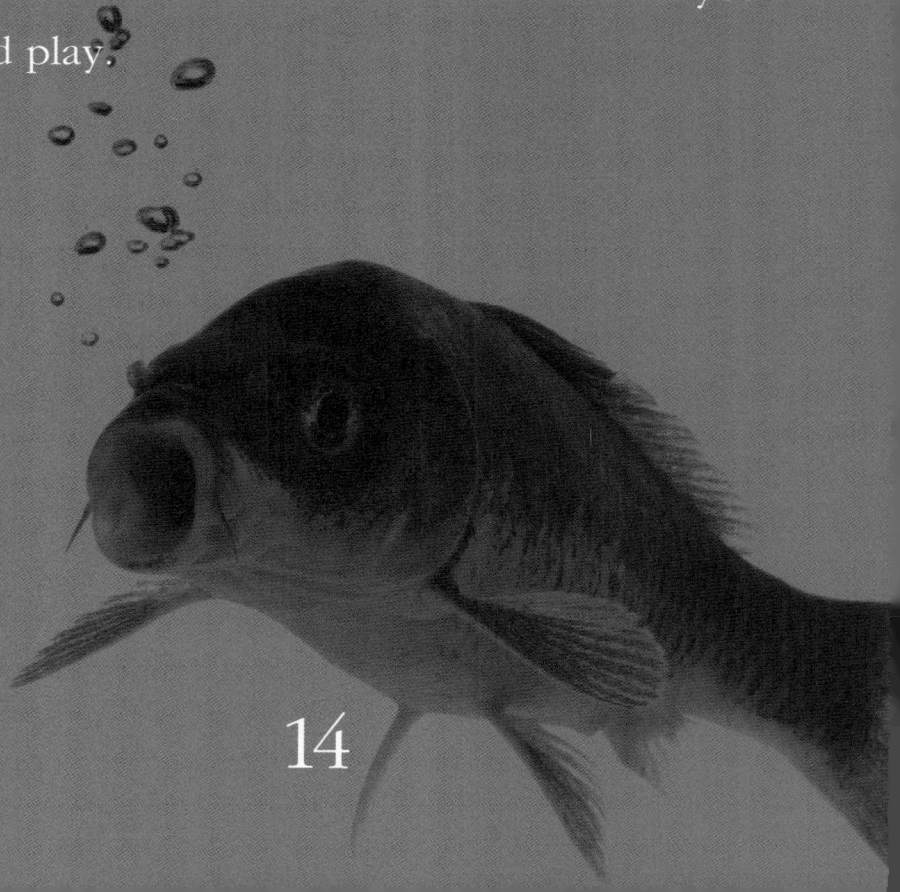

Did You Know?

When you're curious about something, you're more likely to remember what you learn.

15

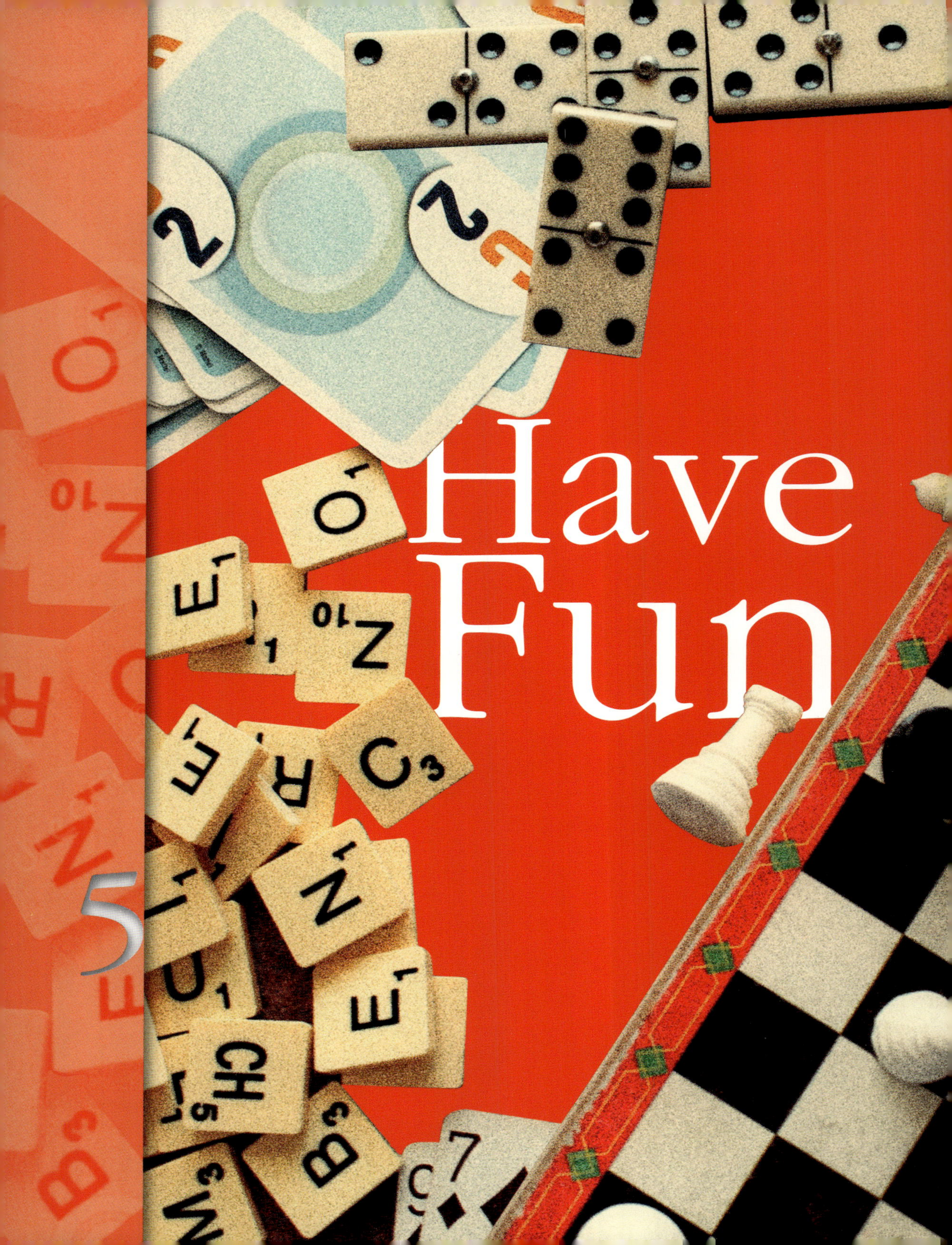

Have Fun

You can have fun and learn at the same time. Playing grows your thinking skills. It gives your brain a workout. You get smarter when you play

When you play a board game, your brain is solving problems. When you play hopscotch or four square, your brain is working to make your body move correctly. When you make art, you exercise your imagination.

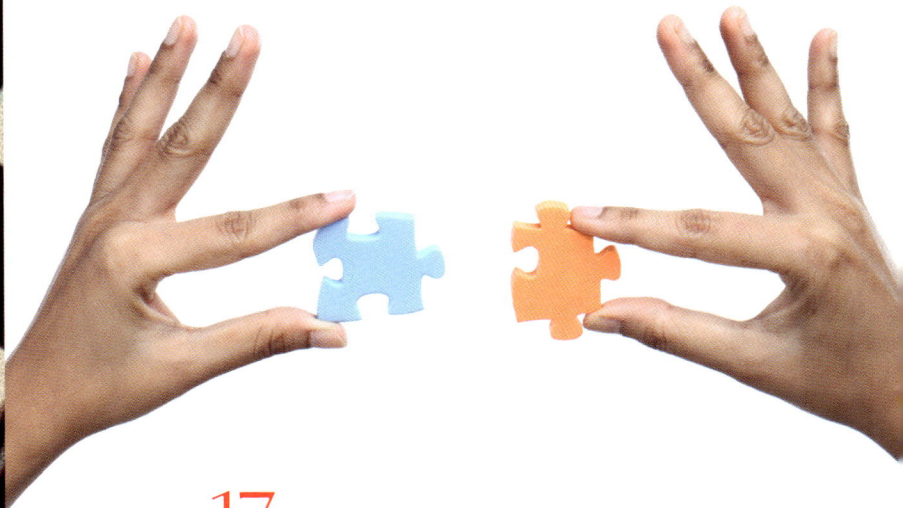

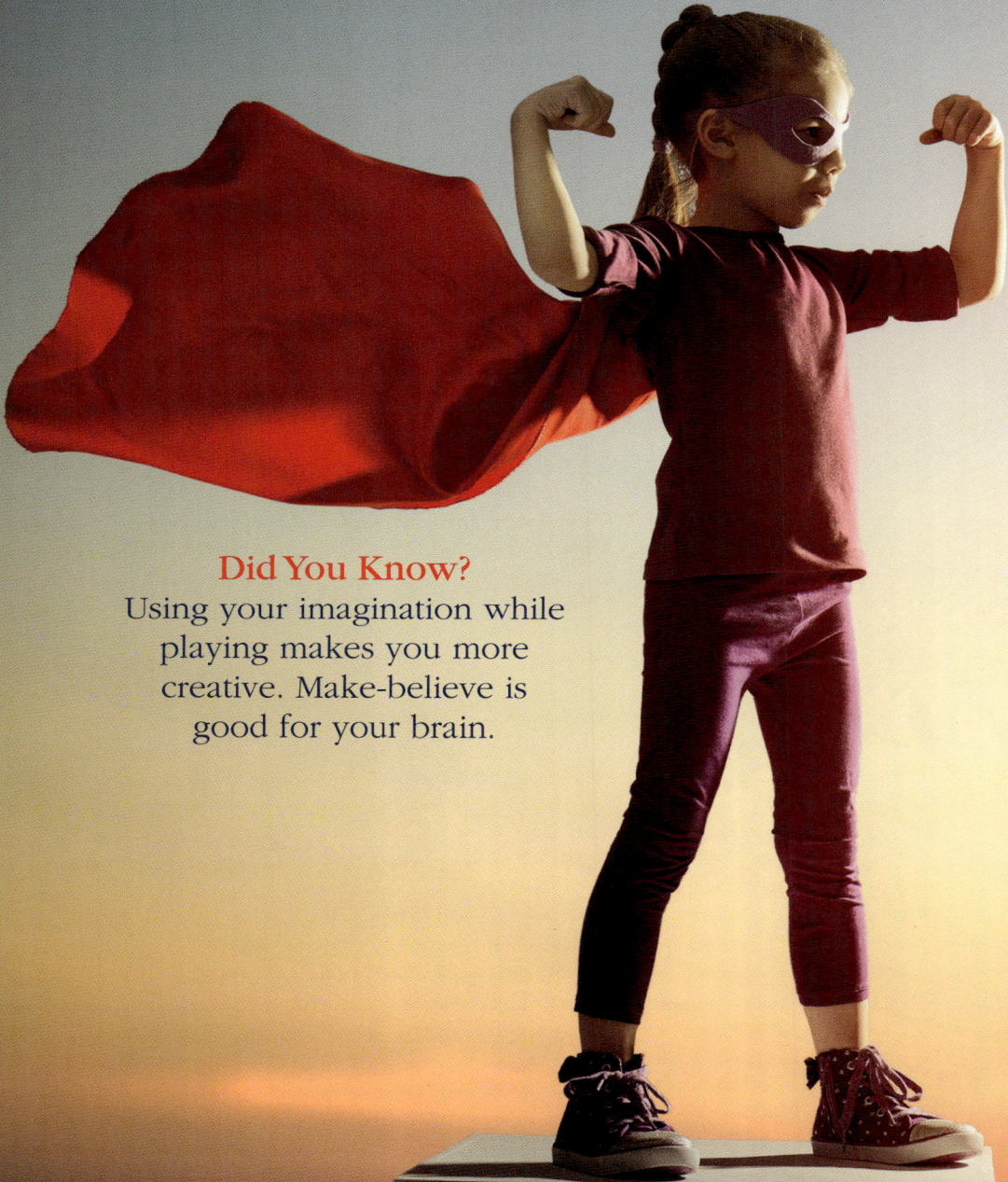

Did You Know?
Using your imagination while playing makes you more creative. Make-believe is good for your brain.

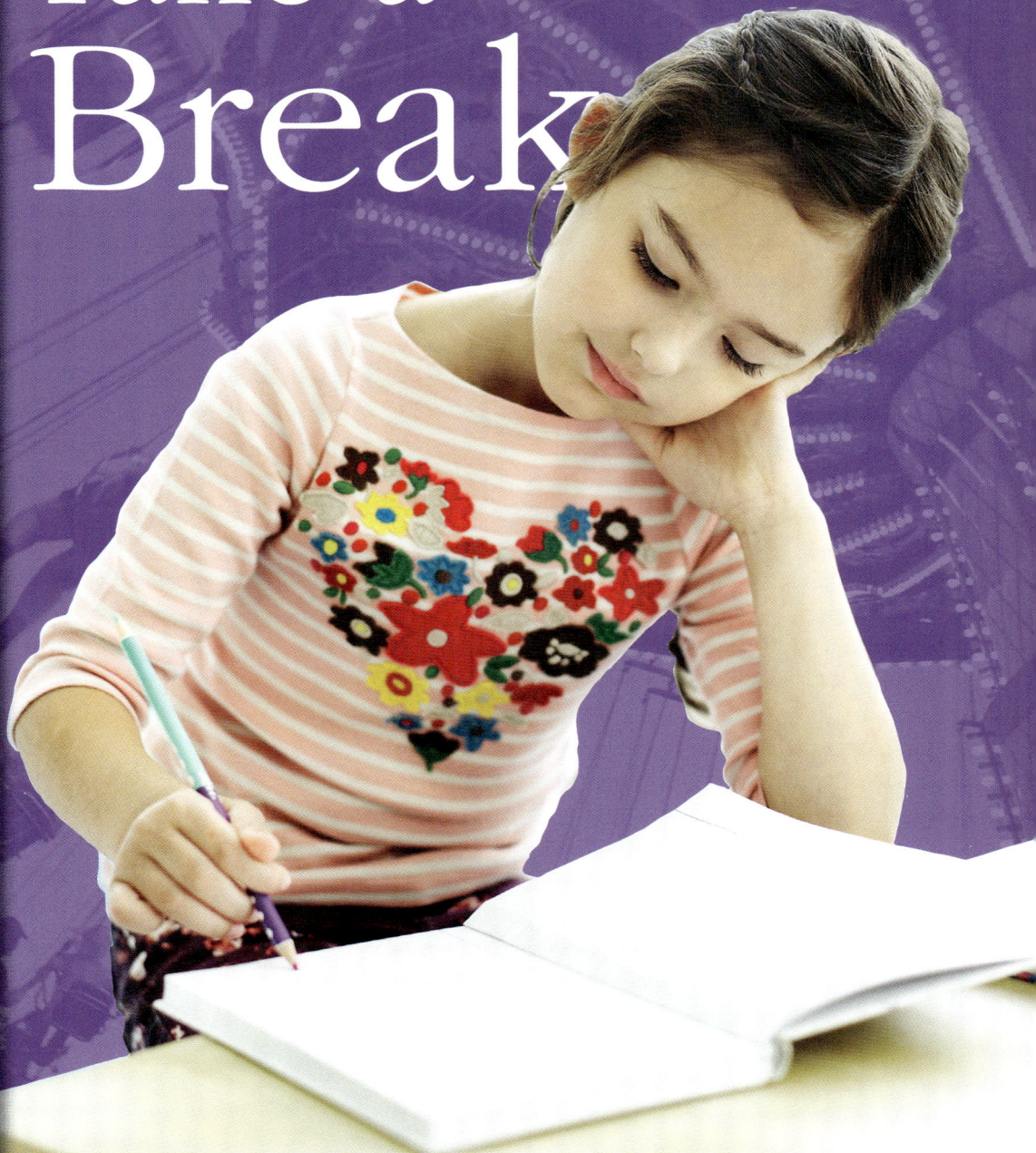

Take a Break

Just like your body, your brain needs quiet time. It needs to unwind and recharge. Writing your thoughts, drawing, or doodling are good ways to take a break. So is daydreaming.

Try to find some quiet time every day. Ten to fifteen minutes is good. After that, your brain will be ready to learn again. Taking breaks might even help your grades.

Did You Know?

Meditation is one way to clear your head. It improves focus and memory.

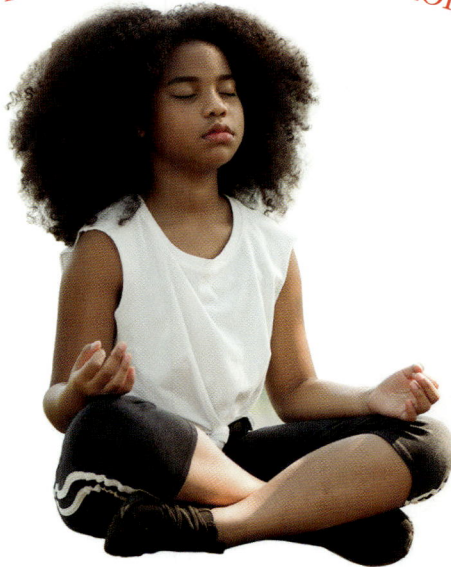

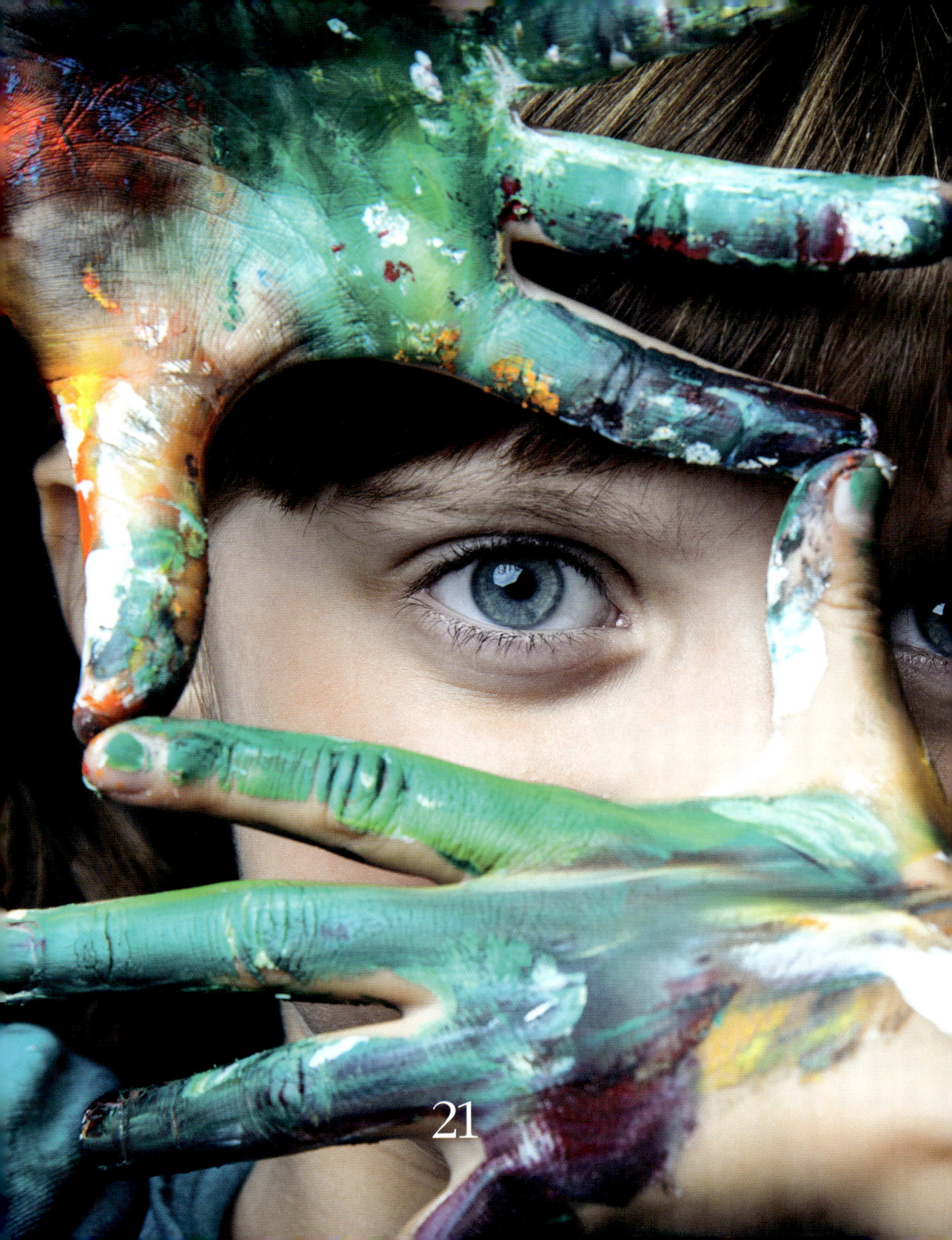

FANTASTIC FACTS

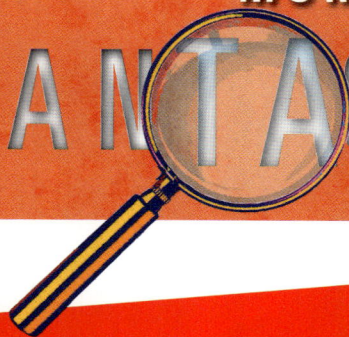

The brain is a wrinkly pink organ.

The brain weighs 3 pounds (1.4 kg). It is 75 percent water.

The brain is protected by the skull. The skull has 22 connected bones.

A child's brain needs 10 to 12 hours of sleep every night. Sleep helps save what you learned during the day.

Brains produce electricity.

It's said that we use only 10 percent of our brain. That's not true. We use 100 percent of our brain.

22

COOL COMPARISONS

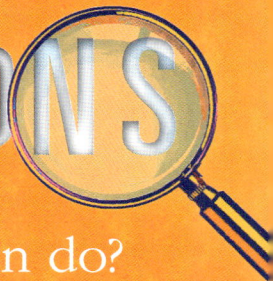

What do the 6 different parts of the brain do?

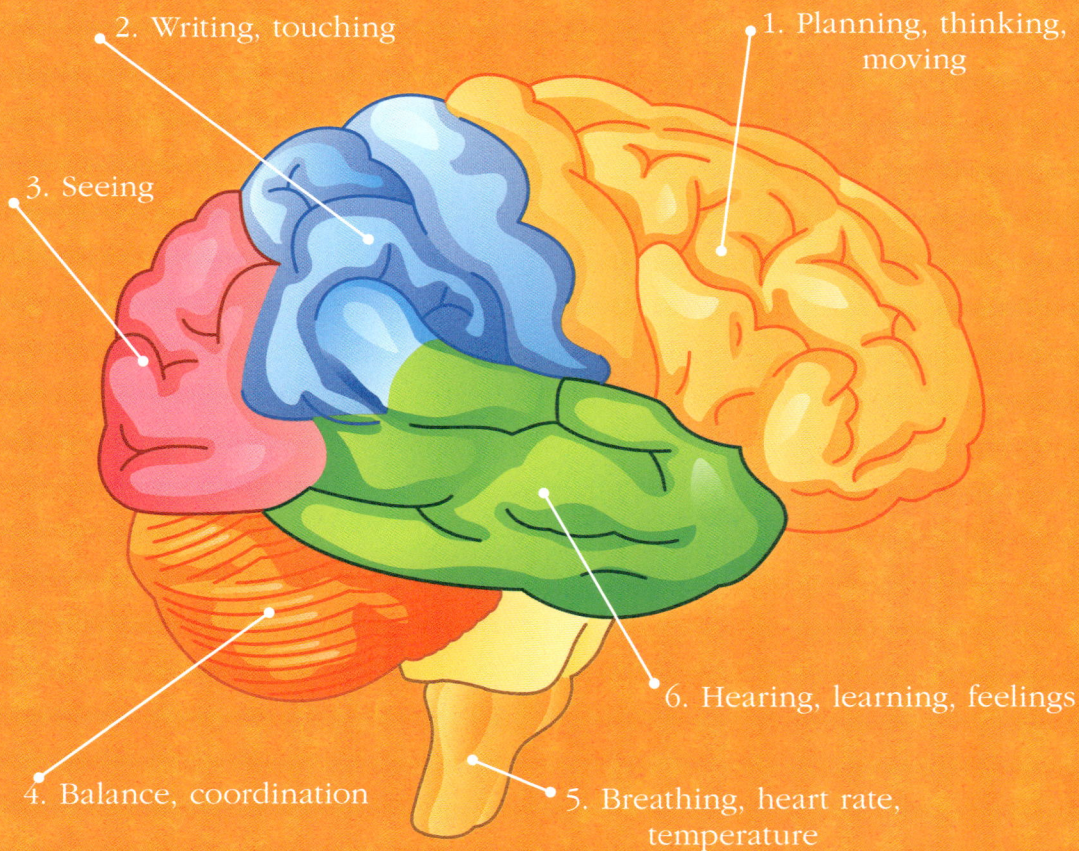

2. Writing, touching

1. Planning, thinking, moving

3. Seeing

6. Hearing, learning, feelings

4. Balance, coordination

5. Breathing, heart rate, temperature

Glossary

fiber (FY-buhr) Plant material that cannot be digested.

meditation (med-i-TAY-shuhn) To spend time in quiet thinking.

mineral (MINH-er-uhl) A substance found in the ground.

process (PRAH-sess) To take in and use.

protein (PRO-teen) A small substance in plant or animal cells.

vitamin (VYE-tuh-min) A nutrient found naturally in foods that is needed in small amounts.

Read More

Hicks, Dwayne. *Your Amazing Brain.* New York: PowerKids Press, 2023.

Lombardo, Jennifer. *What's Mental Health?* New York: KidHaven Publishing, 2022.

Index

curiosity, 14, 15

exercising, 14, 17

nutrients, 11

protein, 11

senses, 5, 23

vitamins, 11, 12

TOP RANK is published by Black Rabbit Books, P.O. Box 227, Mankato, MN, 56002. • COPYRIGHT © 2025 Black Rabbit Books. All rights reserved. No part of this book may be reproduced in any form without written permission from the publisher. • Top Rank is an imprint of Black Rabbit Books. • Edited by Alissa Thielges • Designed by Danny Nanos • Photographs © Dreamstime: Boarding1now, 10, Chrischrisw, 4, Edwin Verin, 6–7, Mariosonic2002, 16, Skypixel, cover; Getty: Alexandra Grablewski 19, Claudia Totir, 12, DEV IMAGES, 17, eranicle, cover, Hammarby Studios, 2–3, miriam-doerr, 11, monkeybusinessimages, 15, PeopleImages, 8–9, Richard Sharrocks, 5, Thomas Jackson, 13; Shutterstock: Amorn Suriyan, 20, Annette Shaff, 19, Eric Isselee, 14, Kuttelvaserova Stuchelova, 21, VectorMine, 23, Yuganov Konstantin, 18 • Printed in the United States of America

Library of Congress Cataloging-in-Publication Data: Names: Snow, Peggy, author. Title: Healthy brain / by Peggy Snow. Description: Mankato, MN: Black Rabbit Books, [2025] | Series: Top rank: healthy and happy | Ages 8–11 | Grades 4–6 | Identifiers: LCCN 2023058218 | ISBN 9781632357977 (library binding) | ISBN 9781645820758 (ebook) | Subjects: LCSH: Mental health----Juvenile literature. | Classification: LCC RA790 .S59 2025 | DDC 616.89----dc23/eng/20240126 | LC record available at https://lccn.loc.gov/2023058218